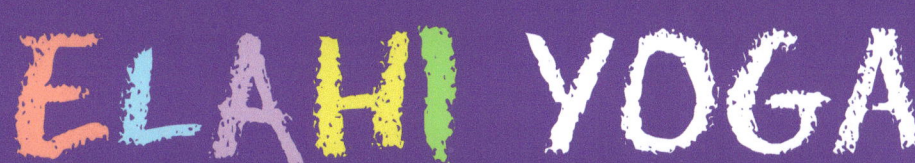

ELAHI YOGA

STUDENT WORKBOOK

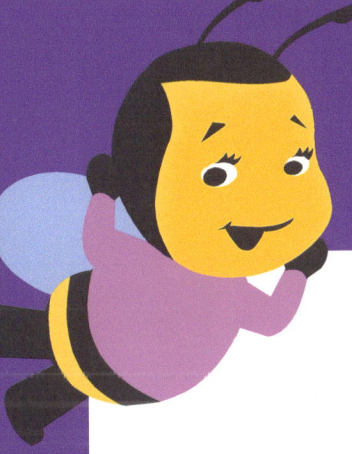

This Book Belongs To:

_____

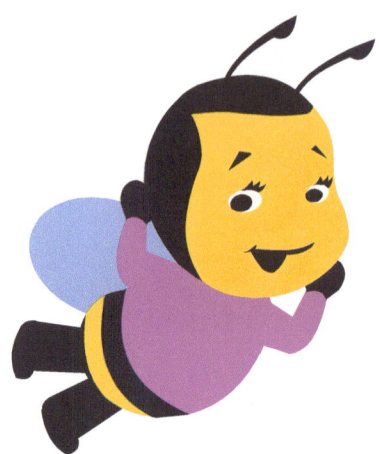

Bee a Yogi!

What is your favorite animal?
Take a photo of you doing
this pose and paste it here!

My name is _____

I am doing the _____ pose!

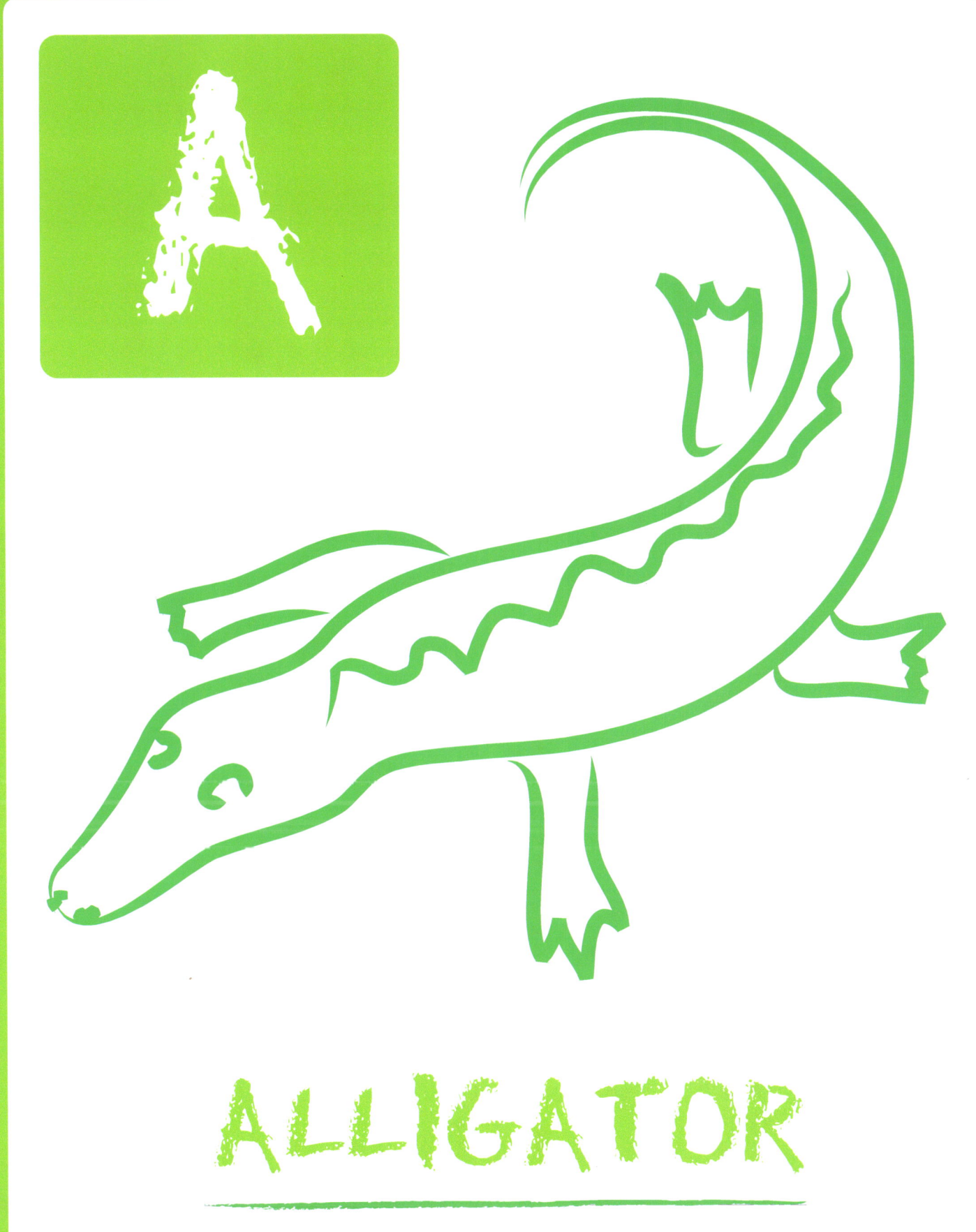

ALLIGATOR

Lay down on your side and CHOMP CHOMP CHOMP your arms together up and down!

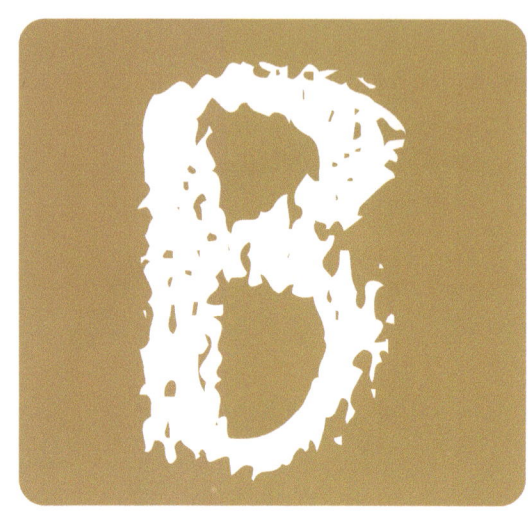

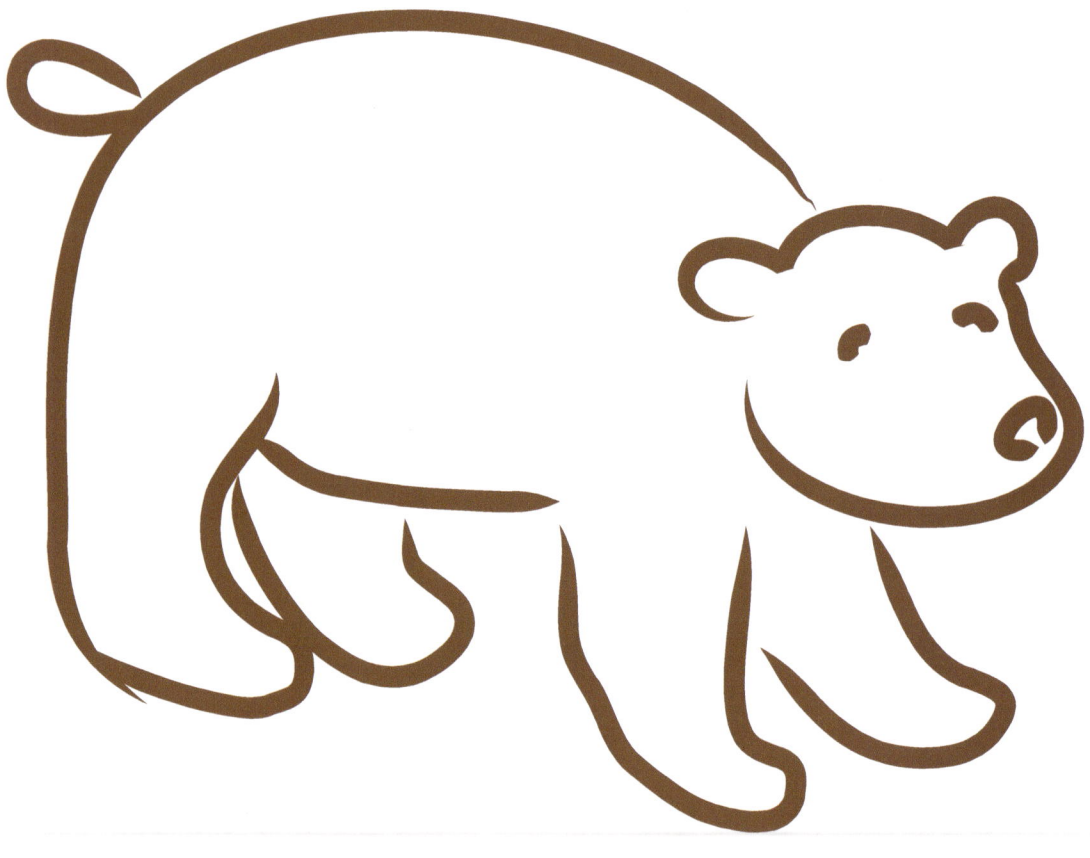

BEAR

Get dow on your hands and feet
and crawl around with your bottoms in the air!

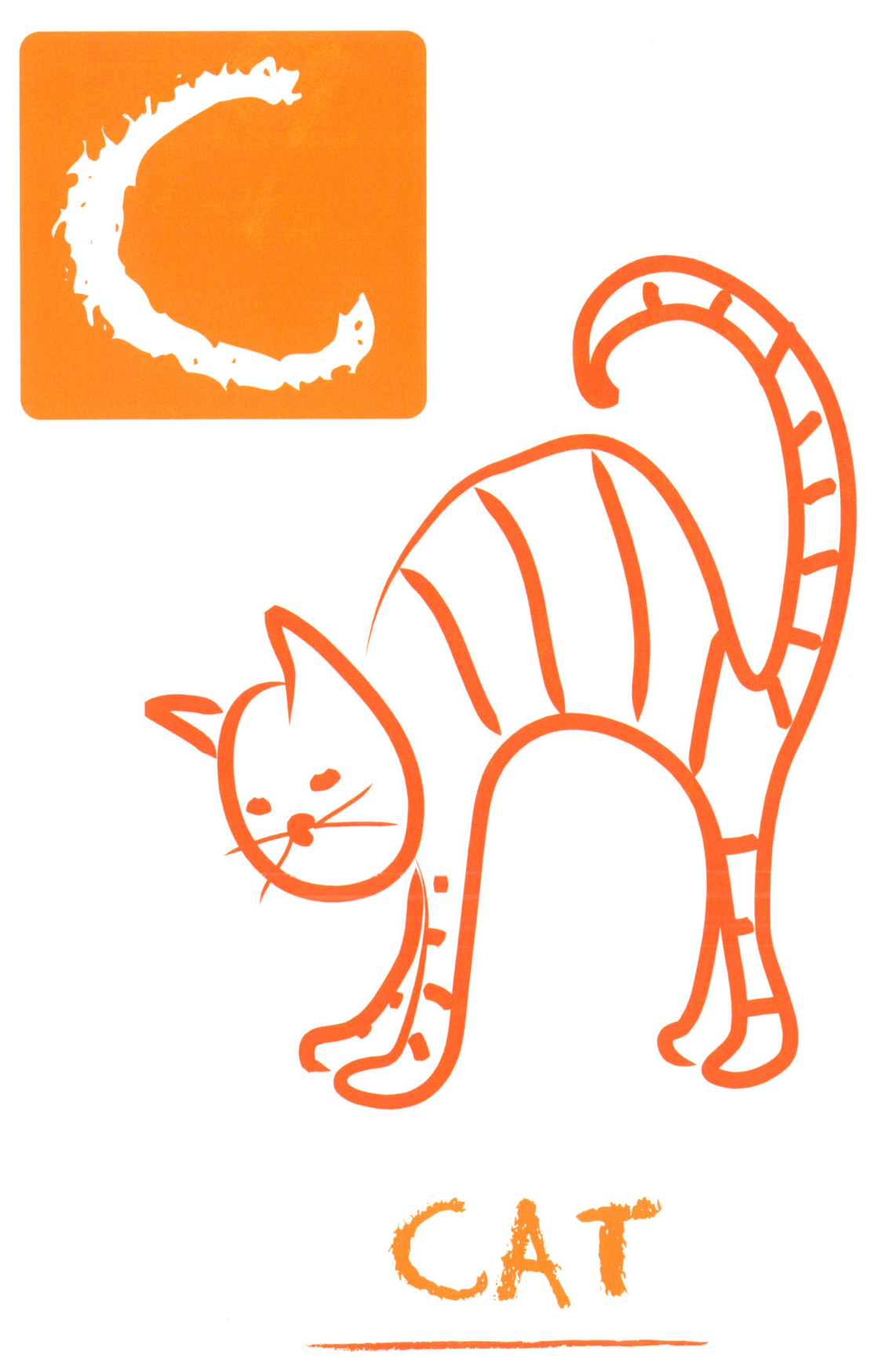

CAT

Get down on your hands and knees and roll your back up to the sky!

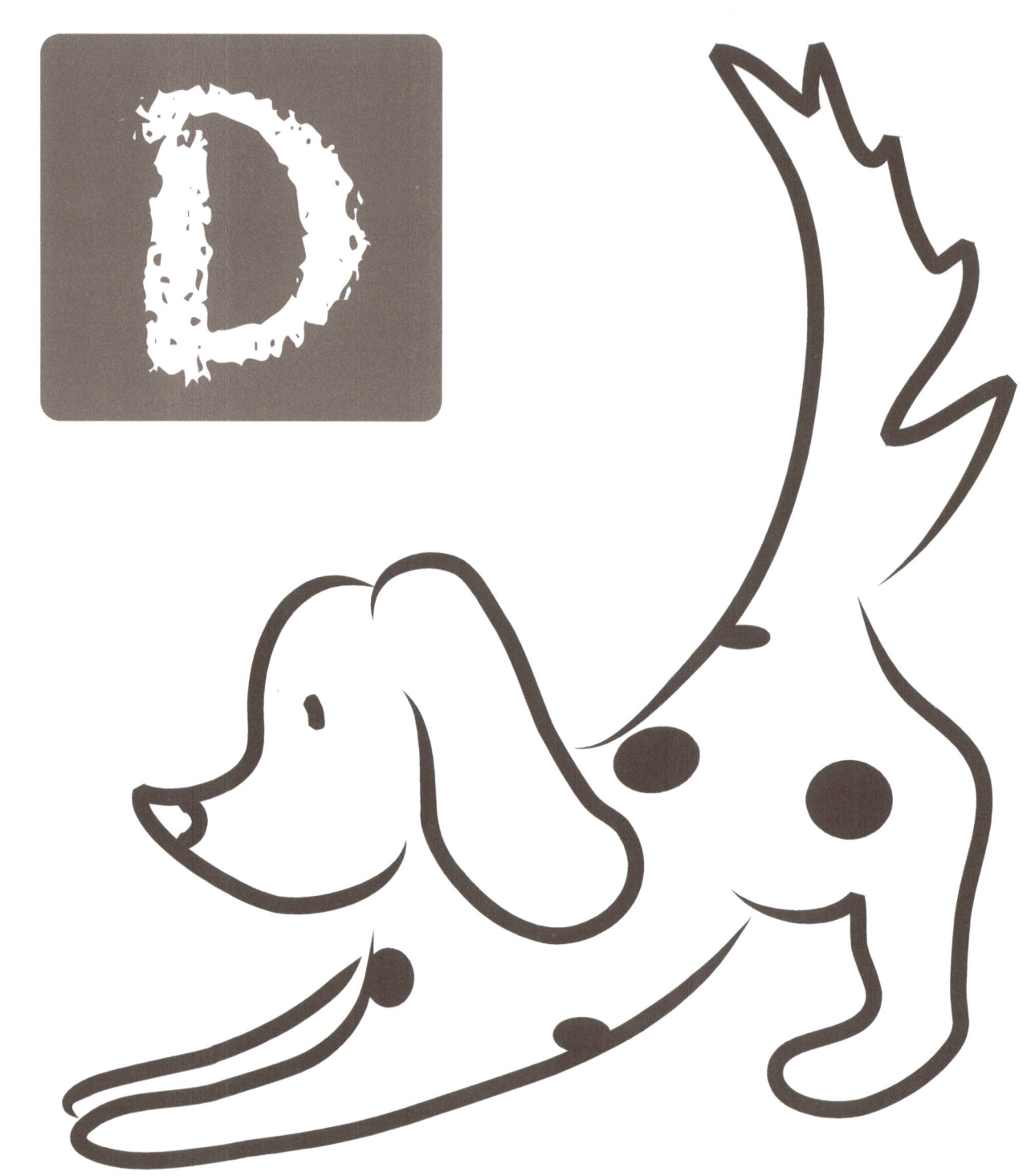

D

DOG

Get down on your hands and feet,
lower your head, and stretch your bottoms up in the air!

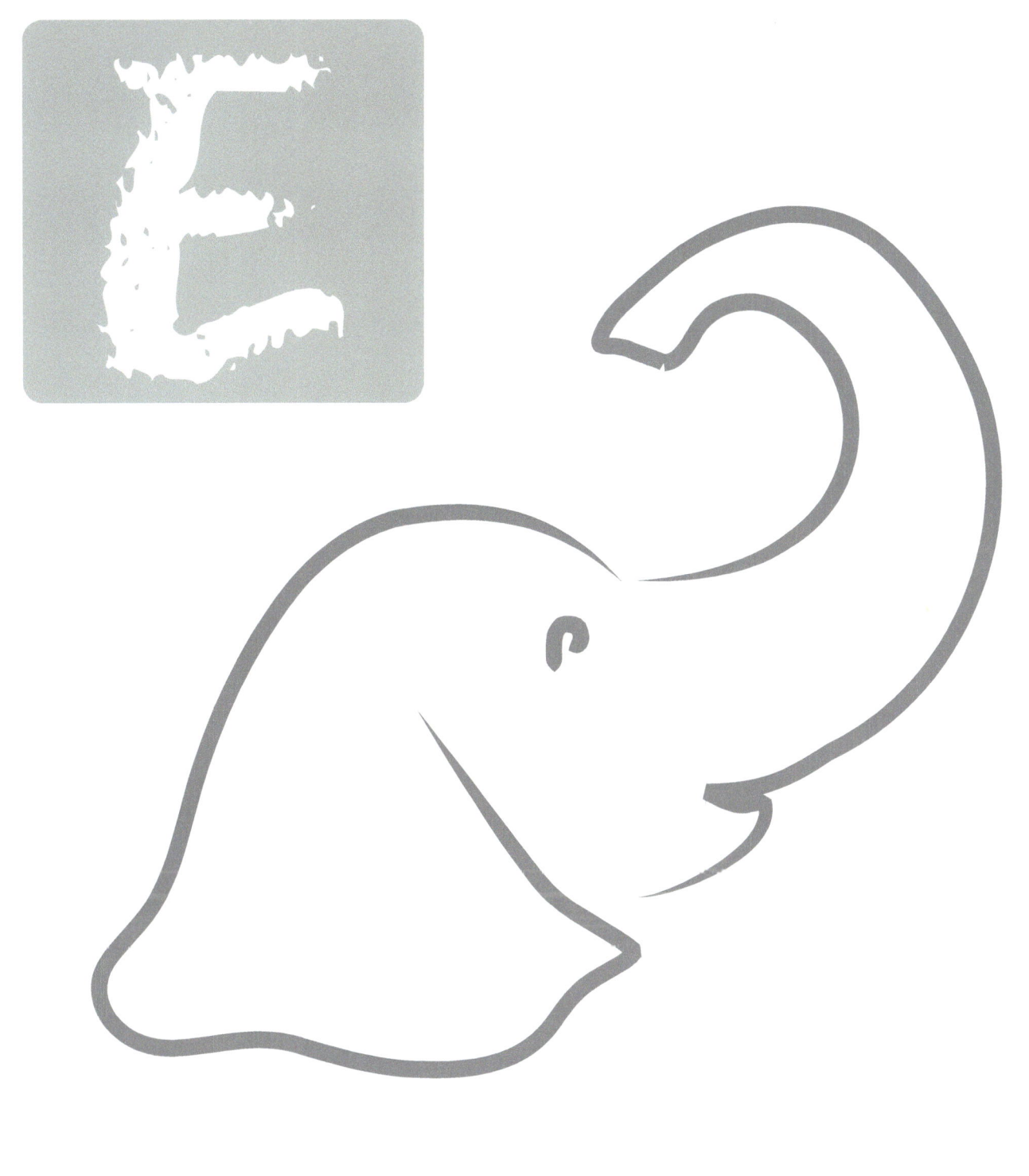

ELEPHANT

Stand up, put your hands together and swing your arms side to side while bending forward to the ground.

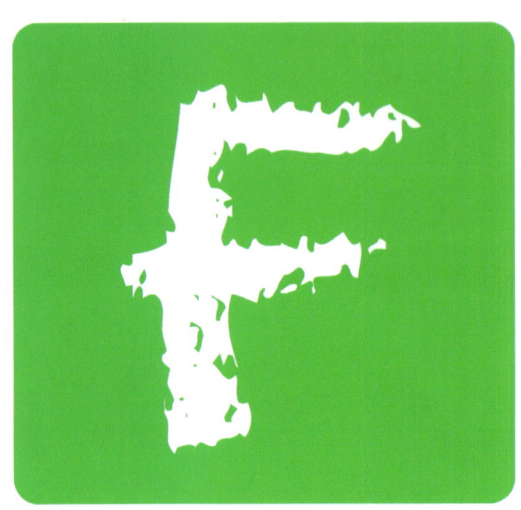

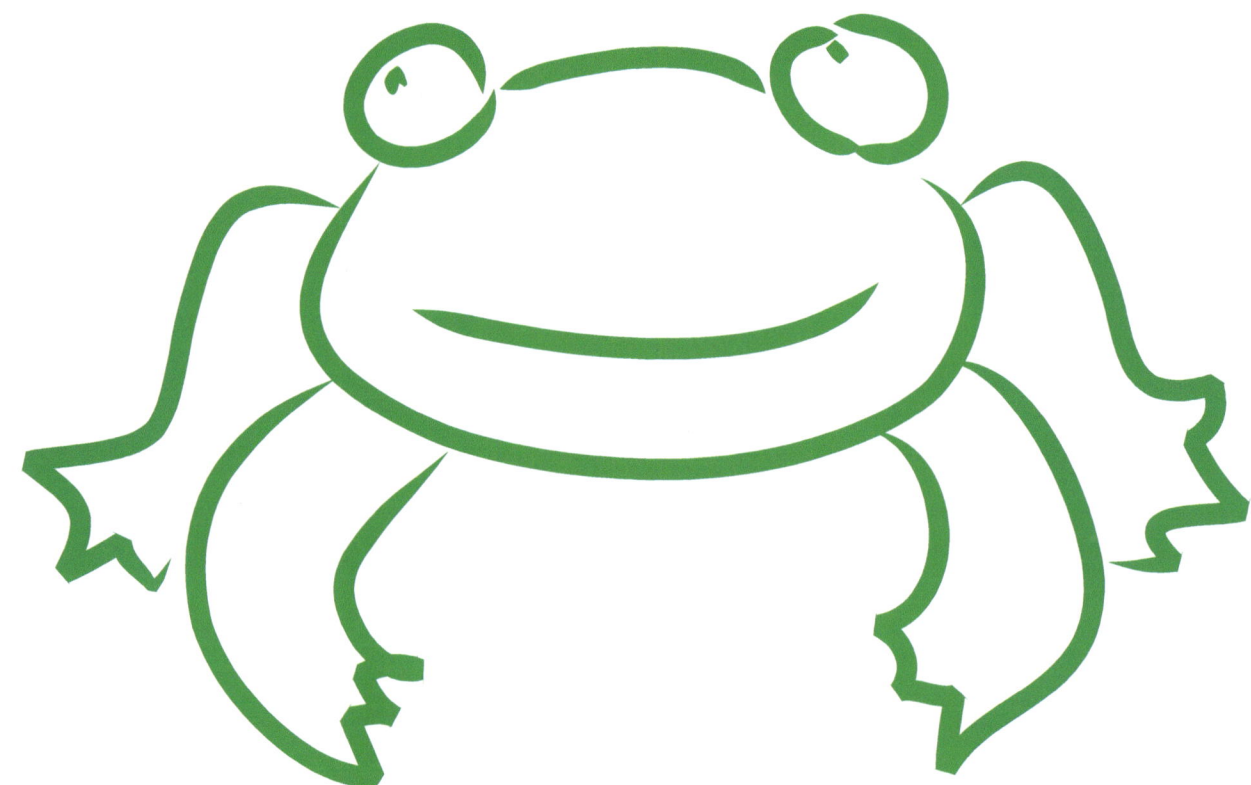

FROG

Squat with your hands on the floor in front of your legs and jump up and down off the ground!

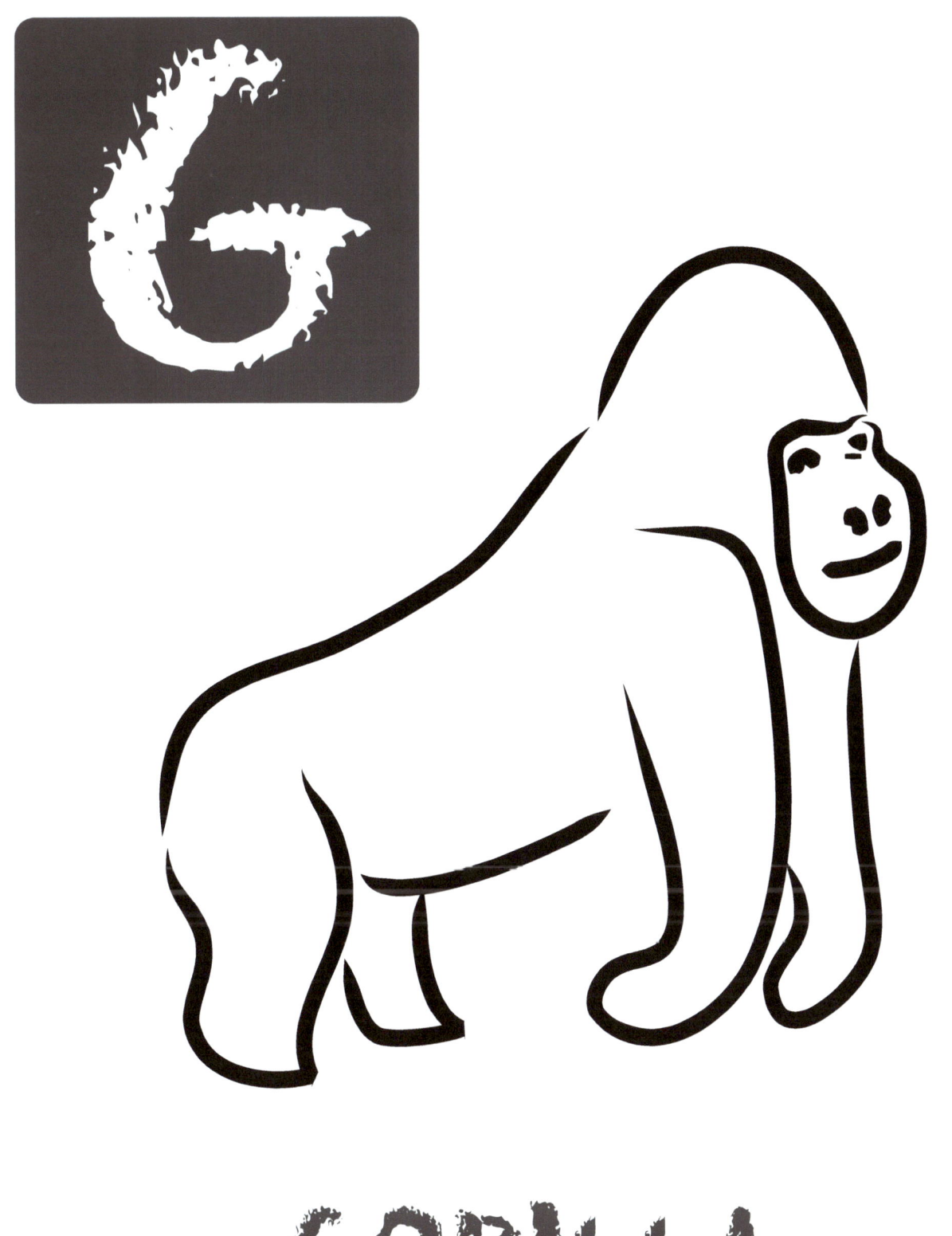

GORILLA

Press your fists into the ground and move your shoulders up and down!

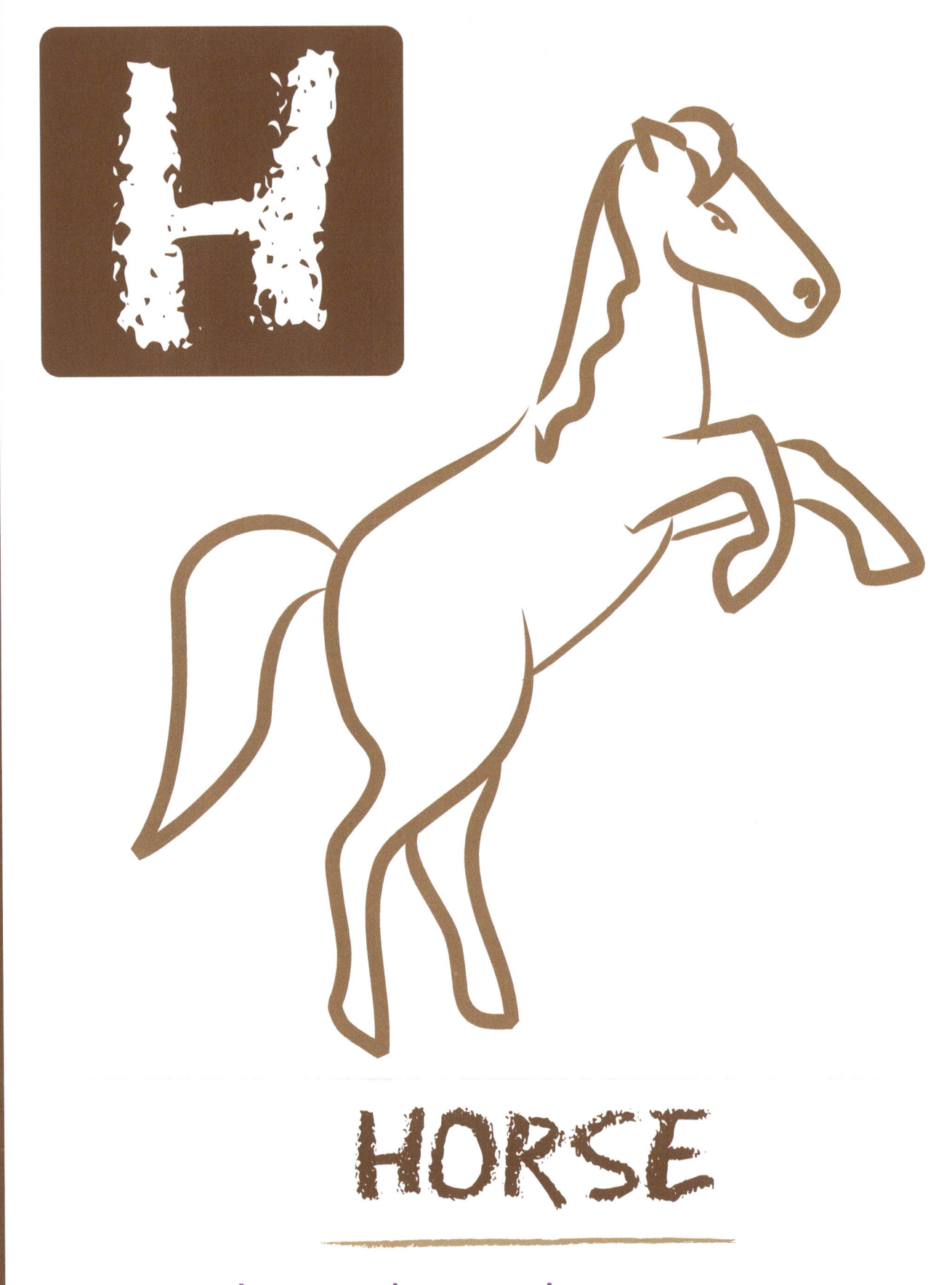

HORSE

Stand on your knees and move your arms up and down in the air.

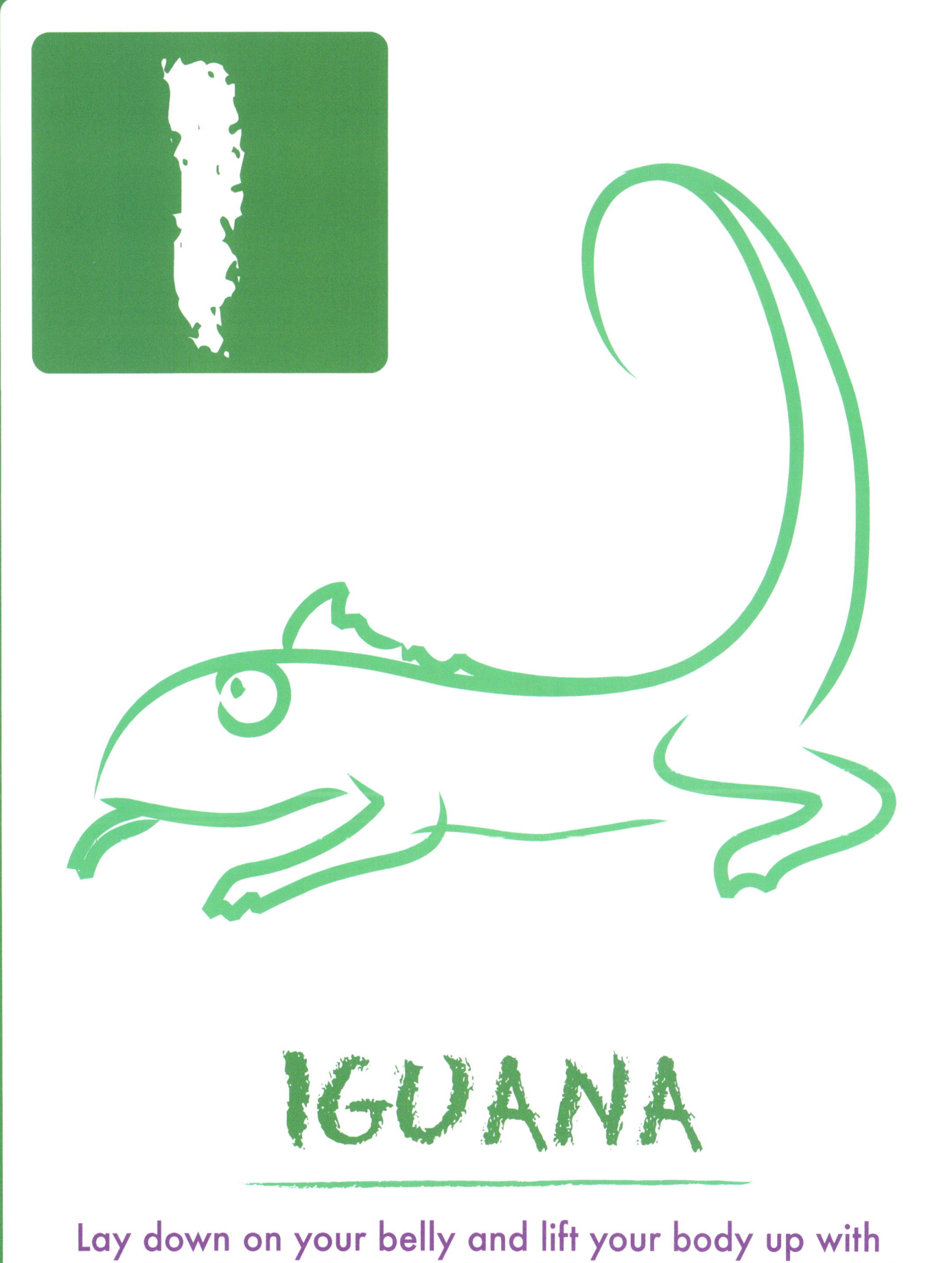

IGUANA

Lay down on your belly and lift your body up with your hands or elbows pressed down into the ground.

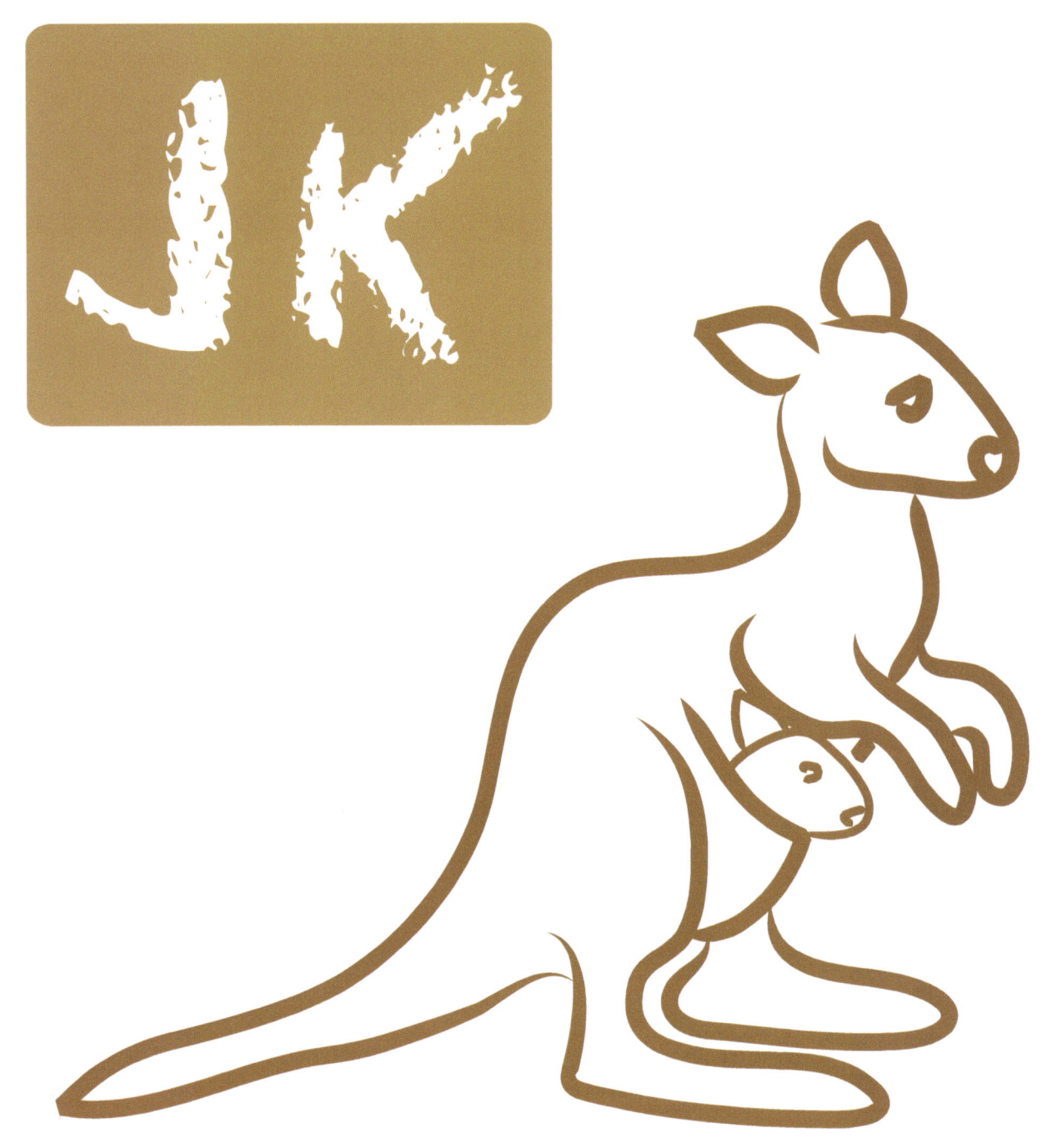

JOEY, KANGAROO

Hold your hands in front of your chest and hop around the room like a kangaroo!

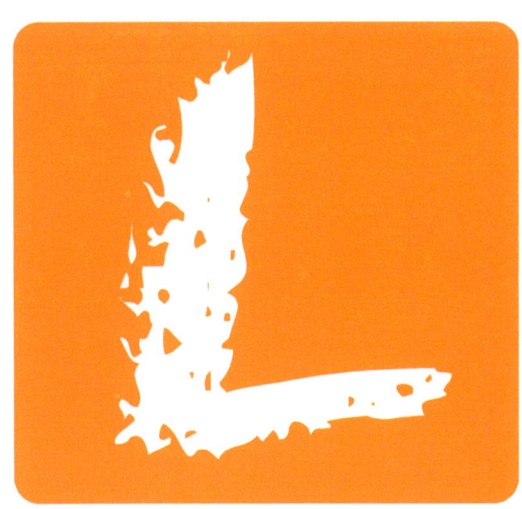

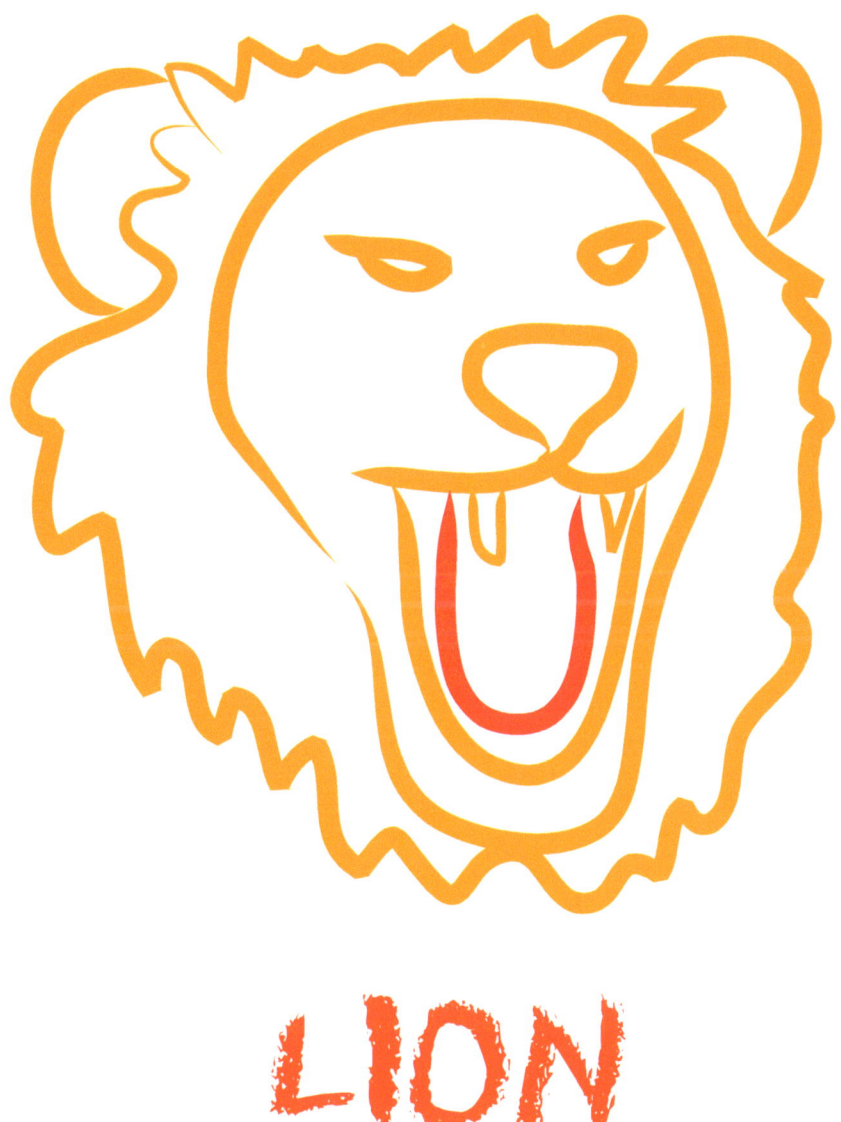

LION

Hold your hands out on each side of your face, stick your tongue out real long, and ROAR!

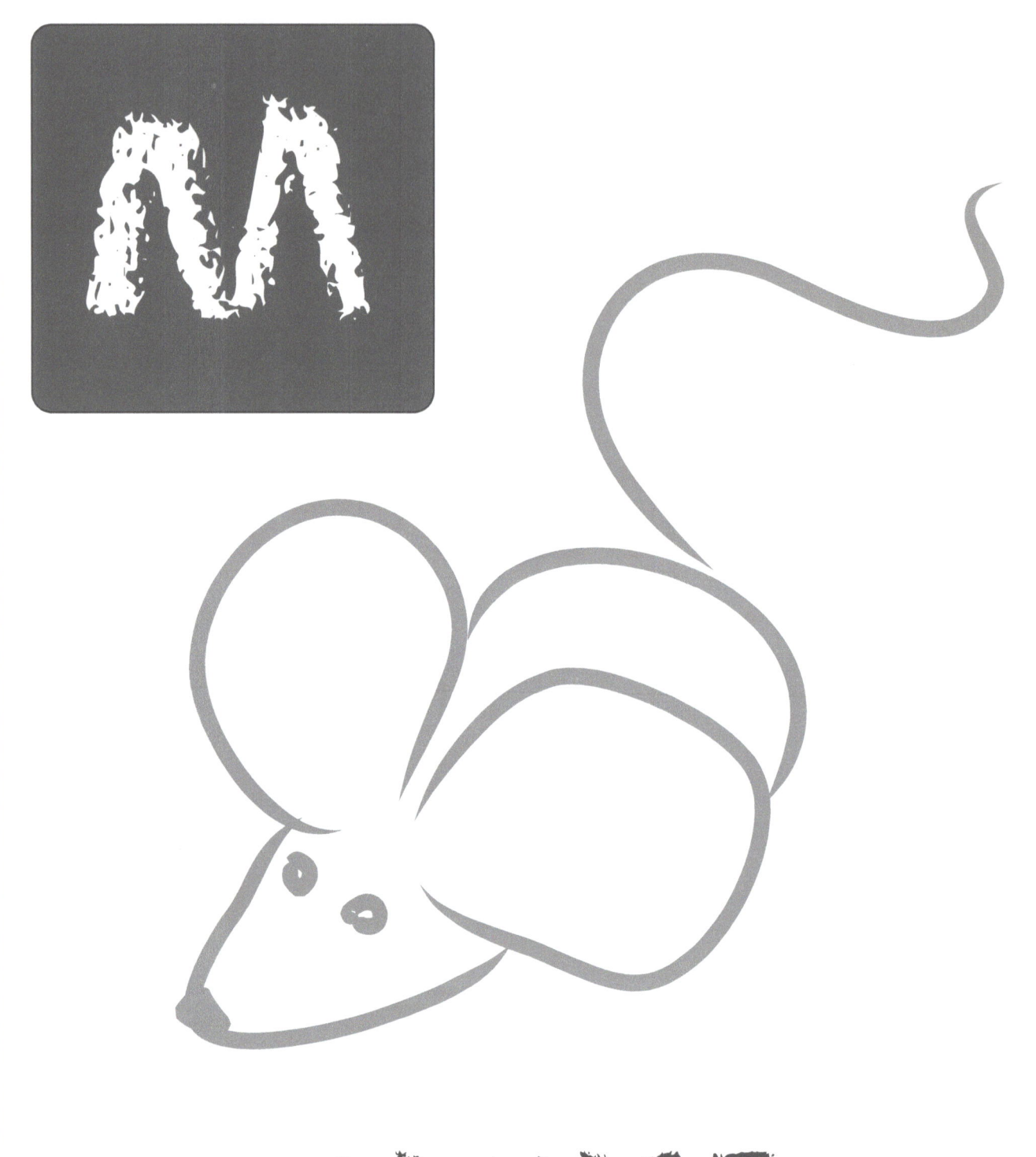

MOUSE

Tuck your knees under your body, put your hands on your sides, touch your chin to your chest, and curl up like a little mouse.

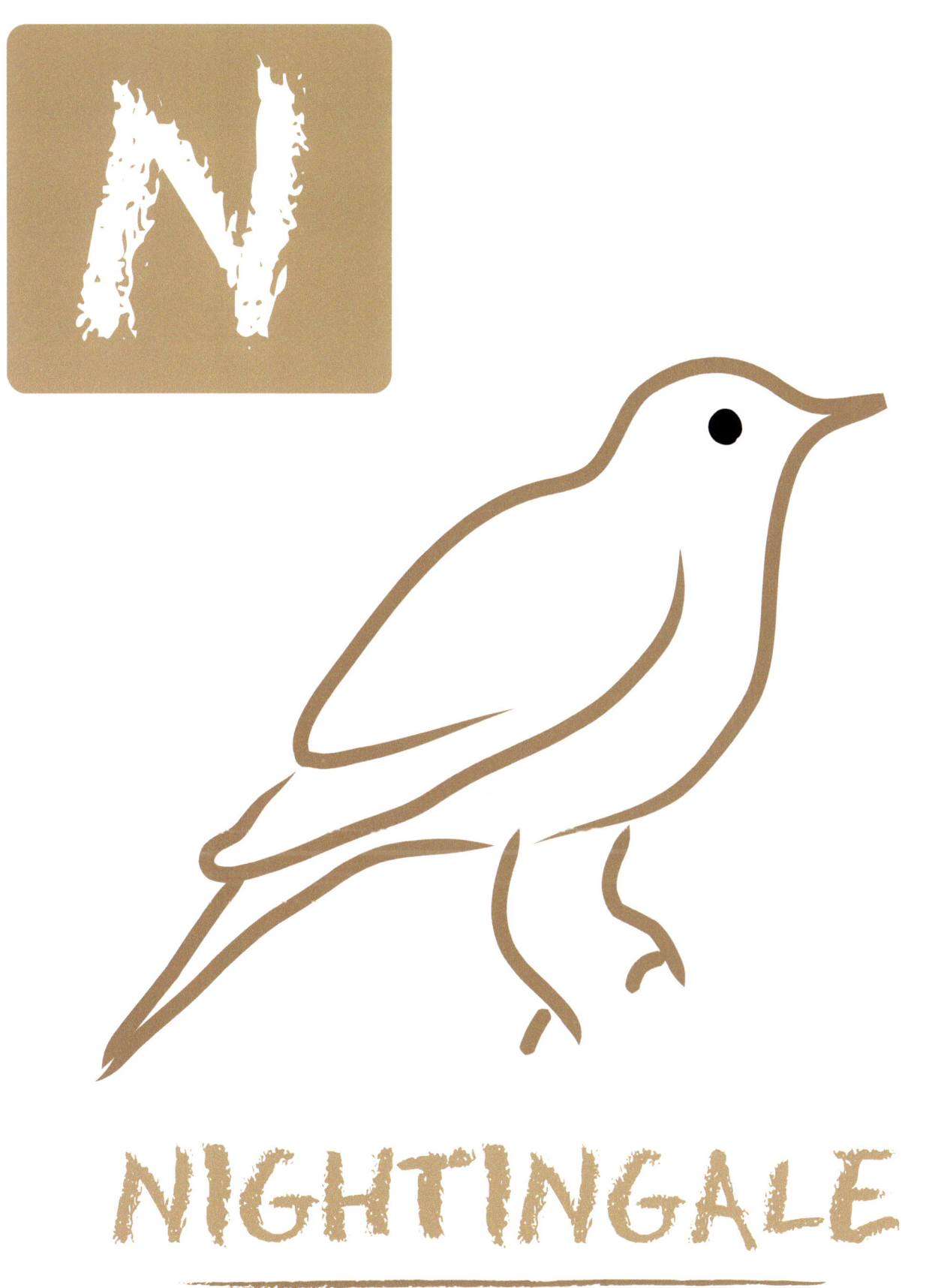

NIGHTINGALE

Flap your arms like feathered wings and soar through the sky like a bird!

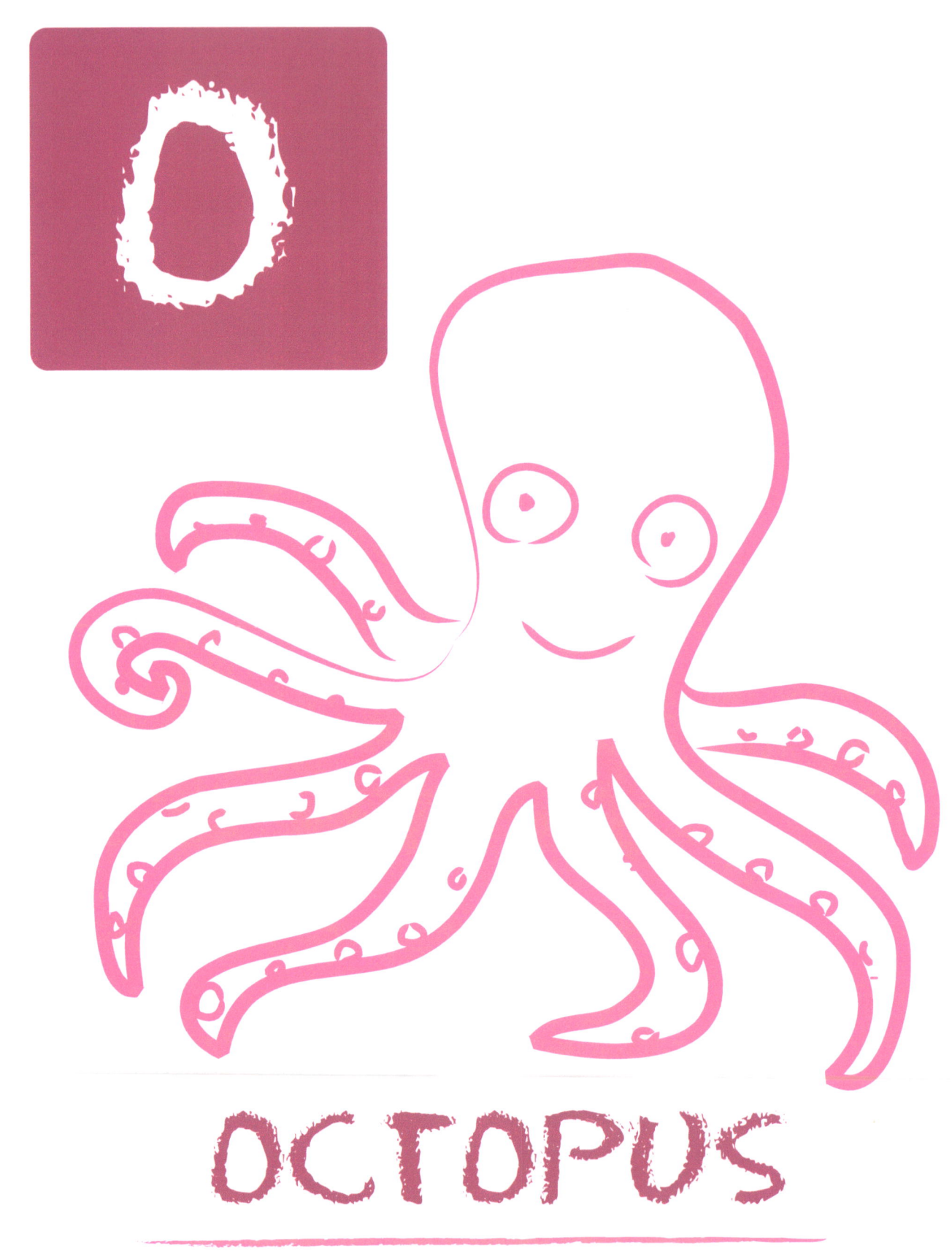

OCTOPUS

Wiggle your arms and legs around your body
like octopus tentacles.

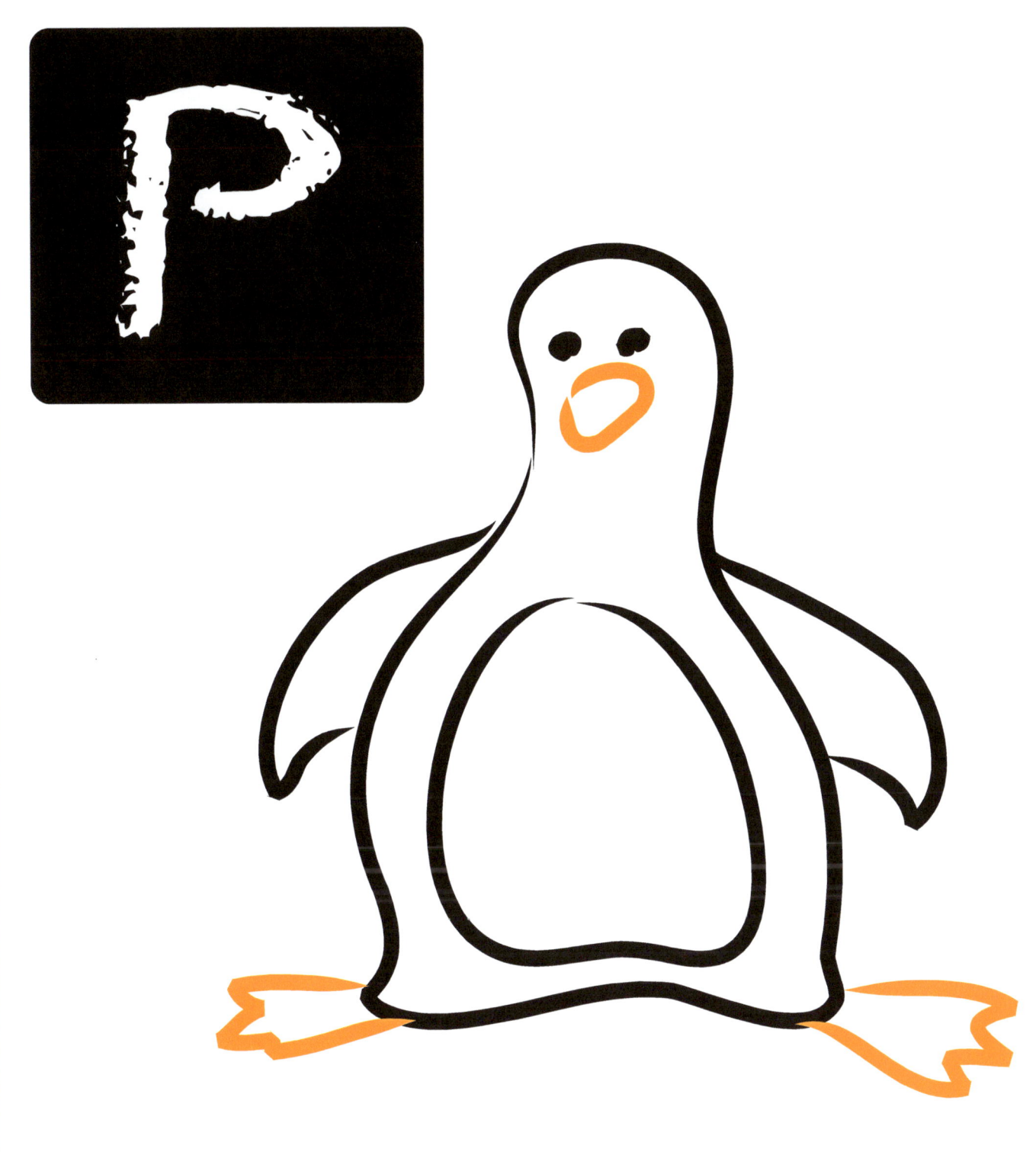

PENGUIN

Keep your legs straight, stick your toes up in the air, put your arms by your side, and waddle around!

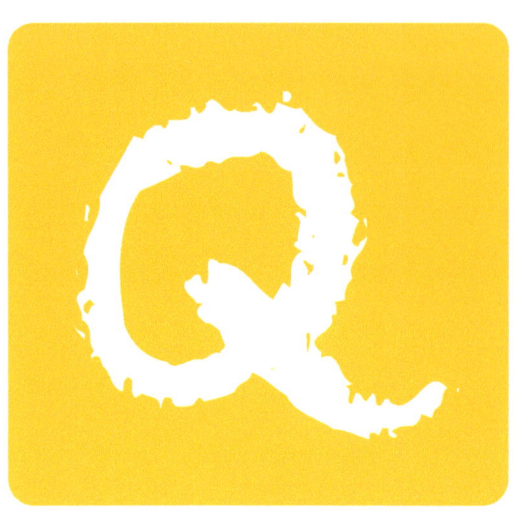

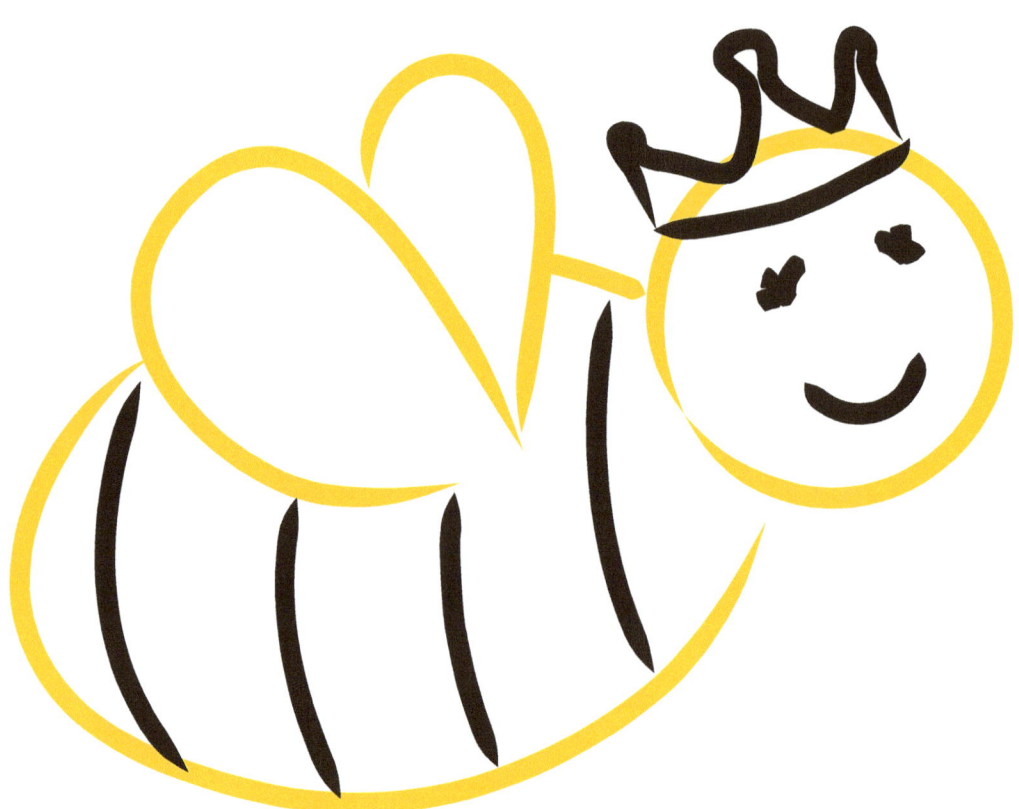

QUEEN BEE

Put your hands on your hips, flap your arms like little wings, and buzzzzzz around like a bee!

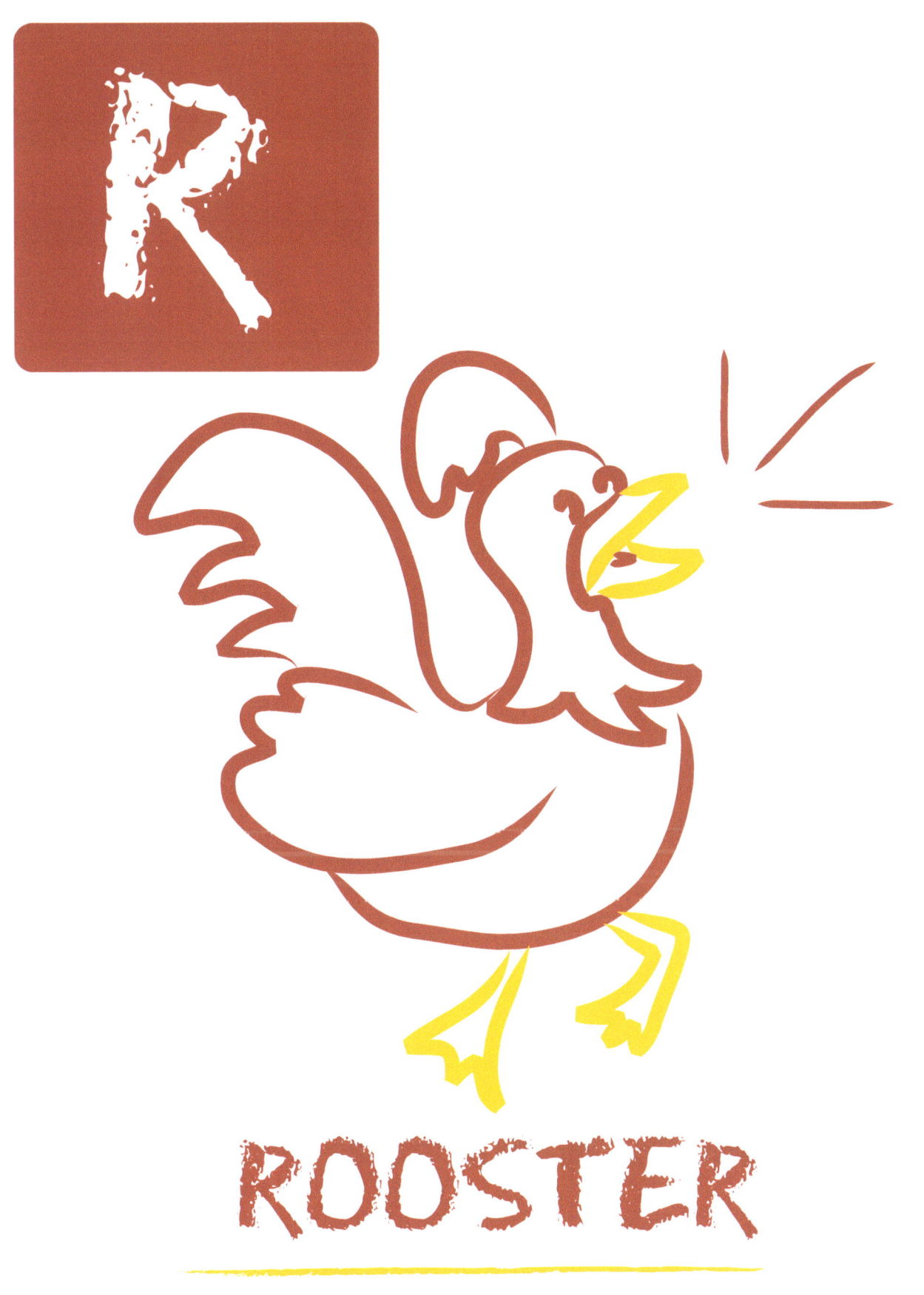

ROOSTER

Hold an imaginary trumpet up to your mouth,
lift one leg up in front, and CROW like a rooster!

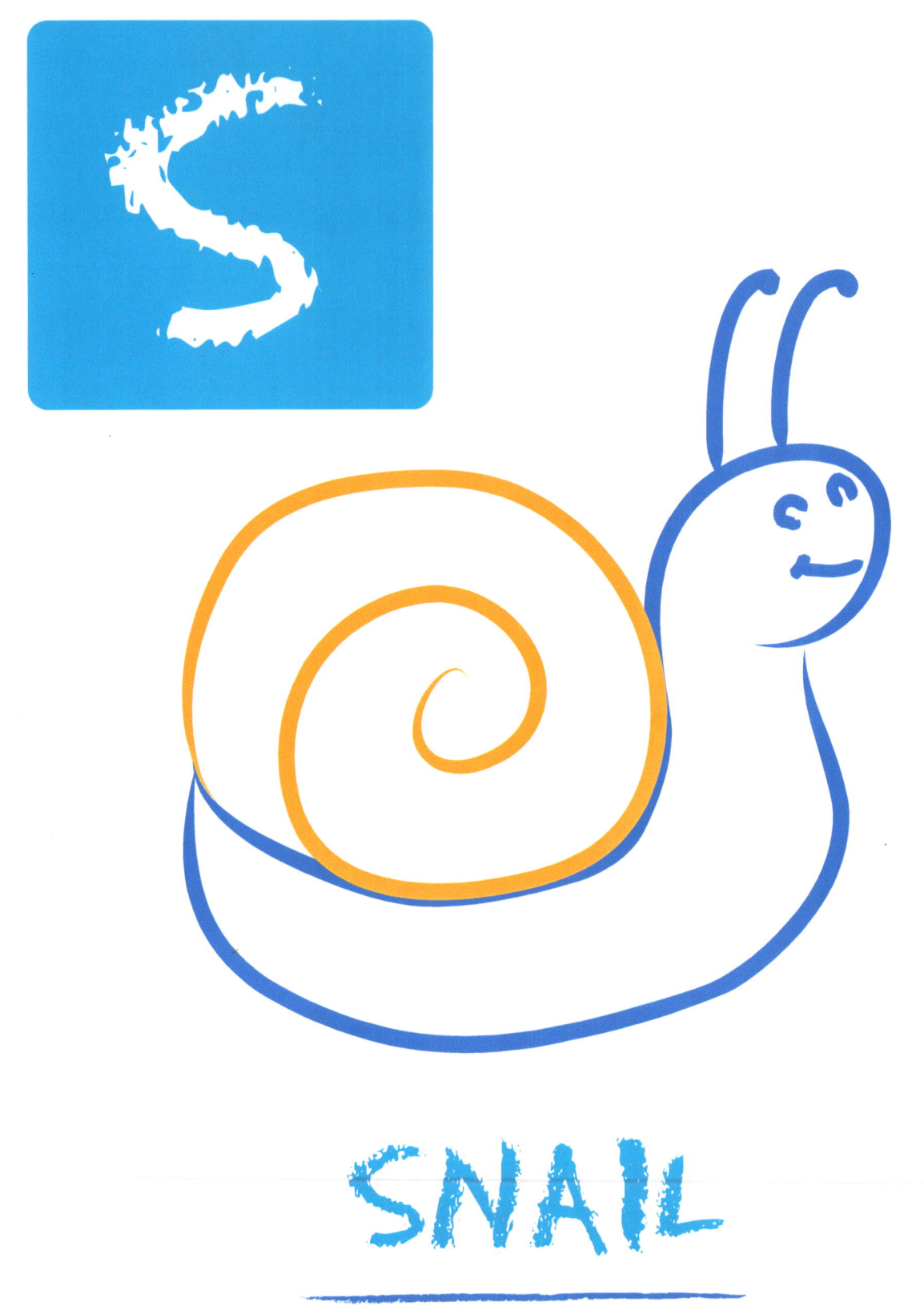

SNAIL

Lay on your back with your arms to your sides, lift your legs up above your head, and touch your toes to the floor.

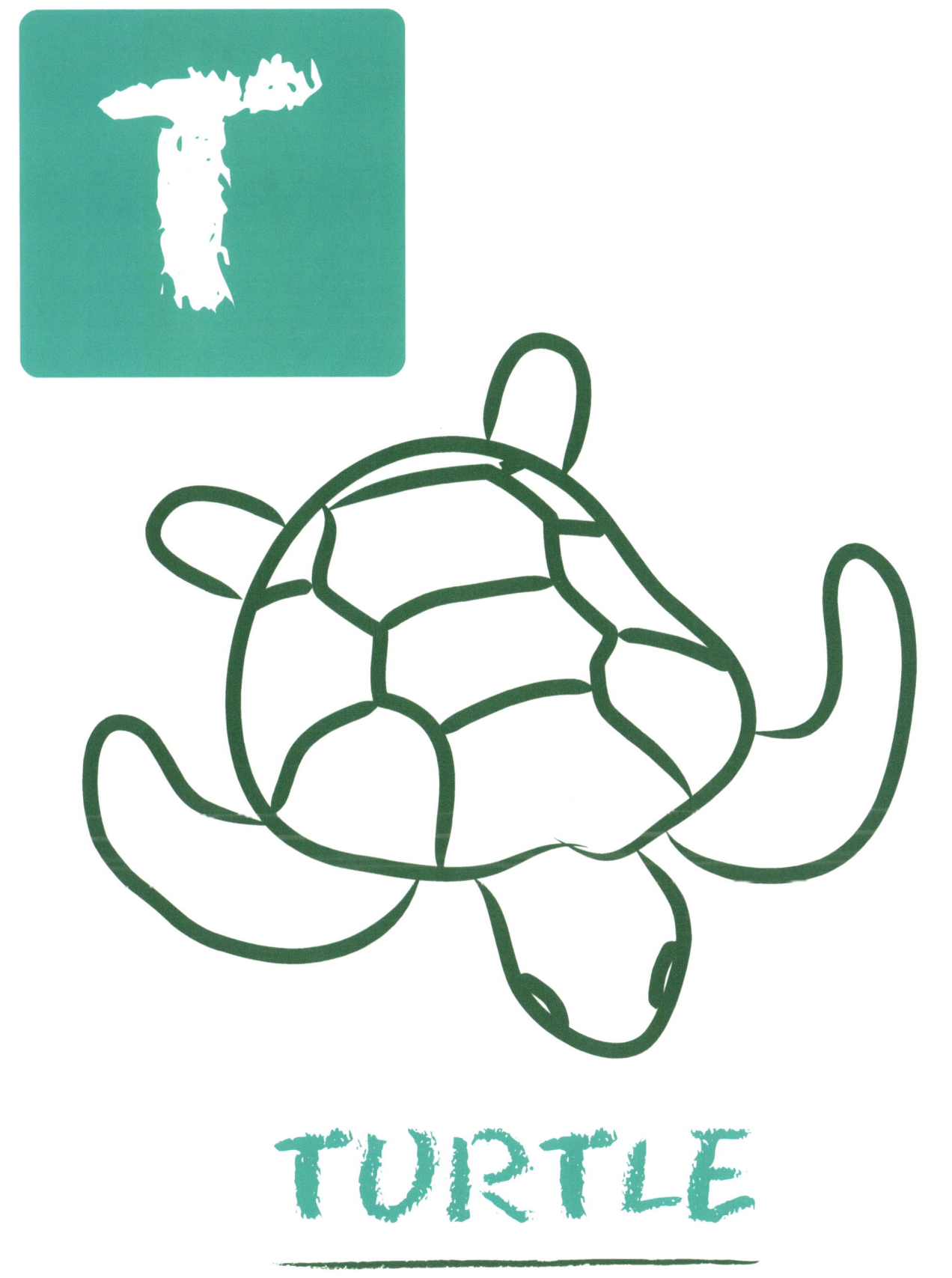

TURTLE

Sit like a butterfly with your feet and toes together, and stretch your hands down under your legs.

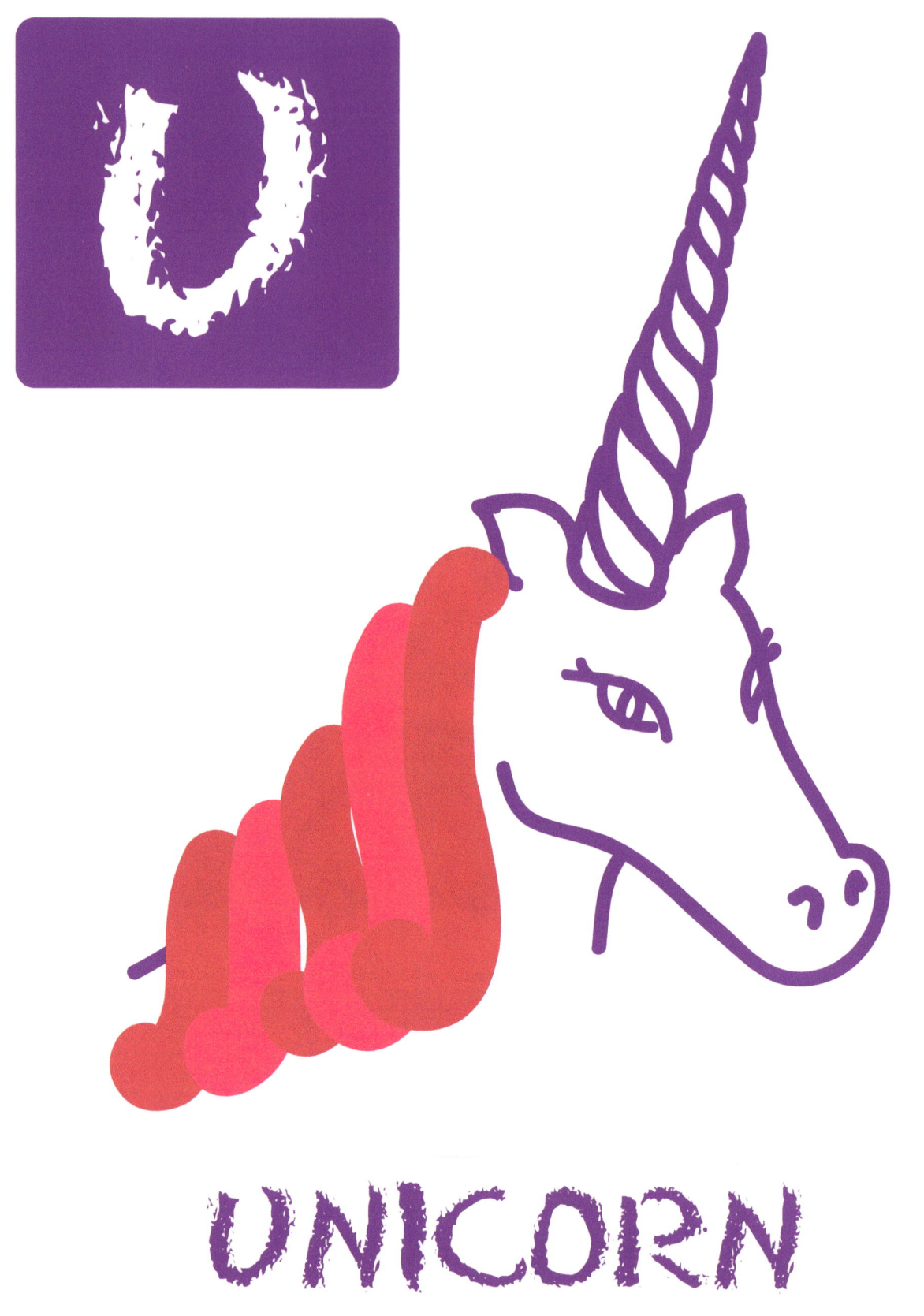

UNICORN

Make a long horn on your head with your arms and trot around the room with your legs.

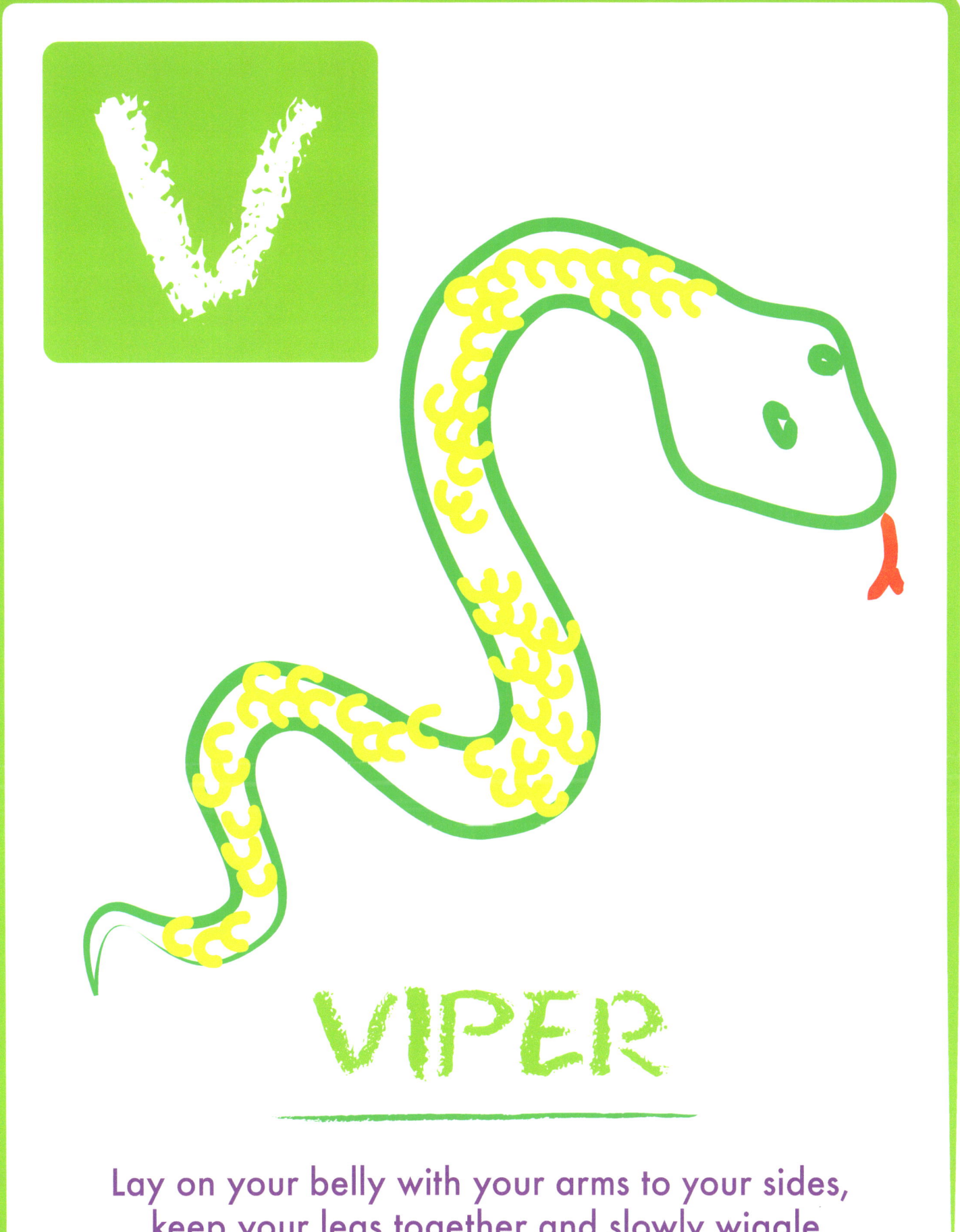

VIPER

Lay on your belly with your arms to your sides, keep your legs together and slowly wiggle your body on the ground and hissssss.

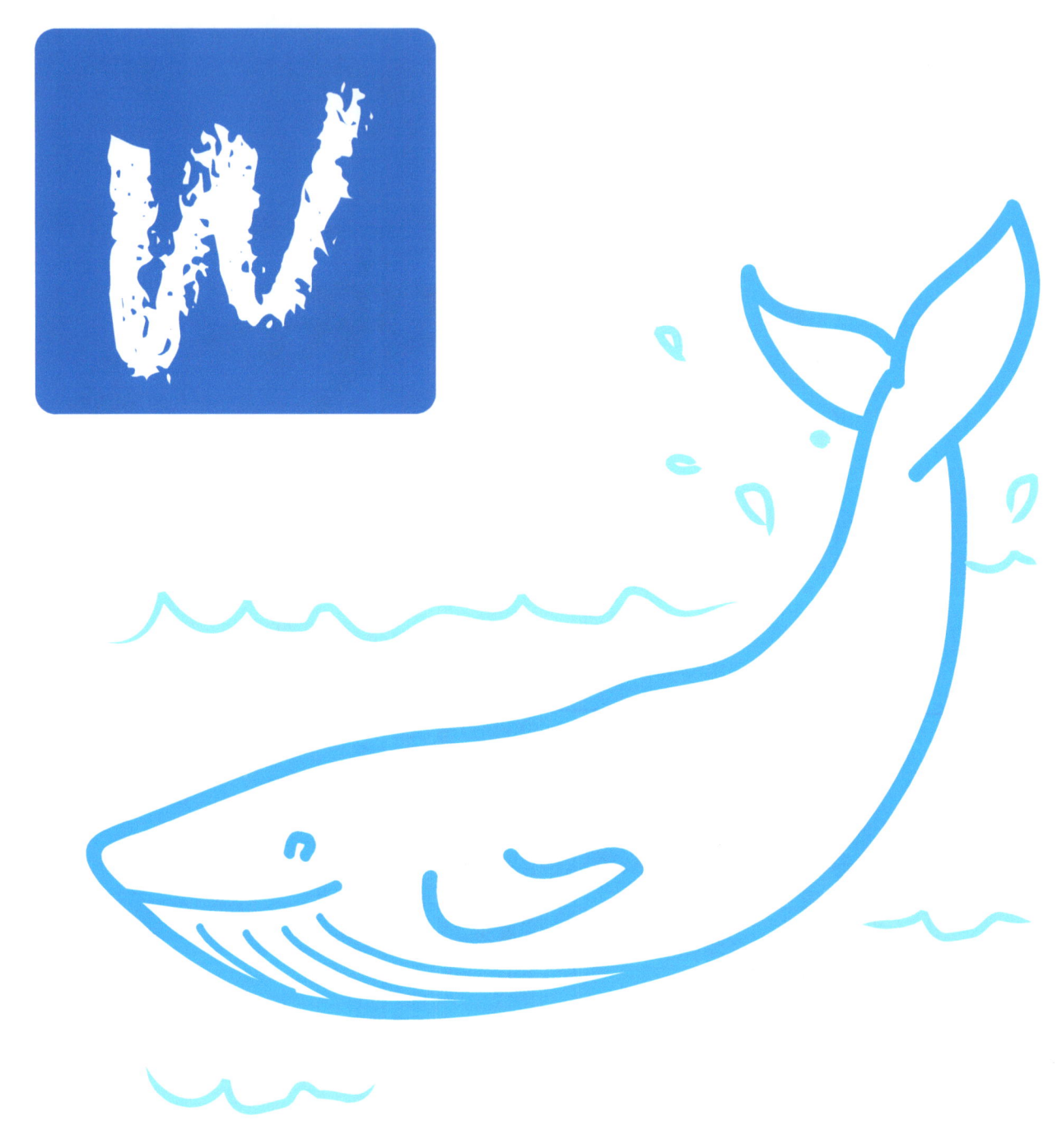

WHALE

Lay on your belly, put your feet together in the air like a whale tail and make a big splash!

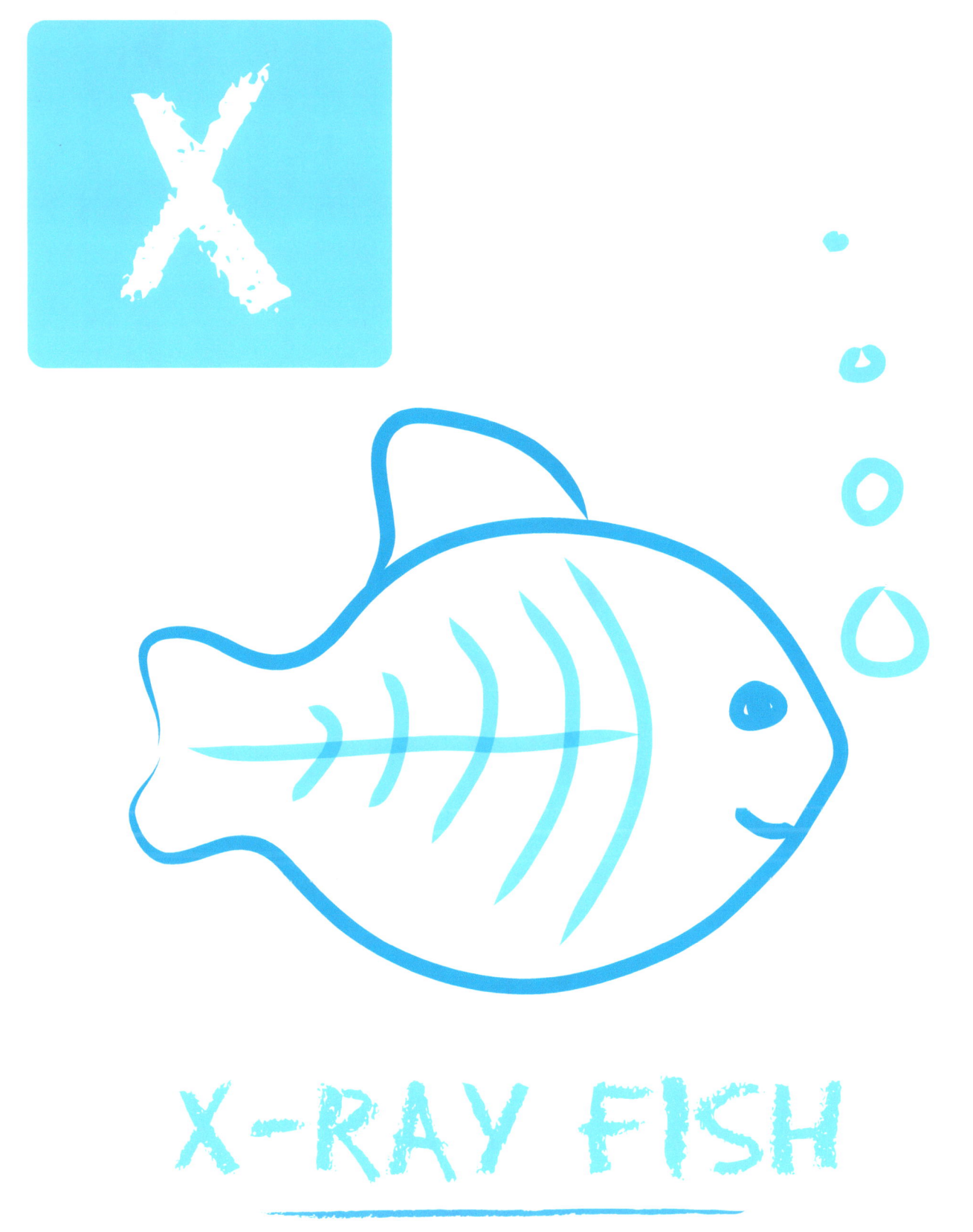

X-RAY FISH

Sit on your bottom, bend your knees and lift your feet up in the air. Flap your hands like fishy fins and make a fishy sound with your mouth!

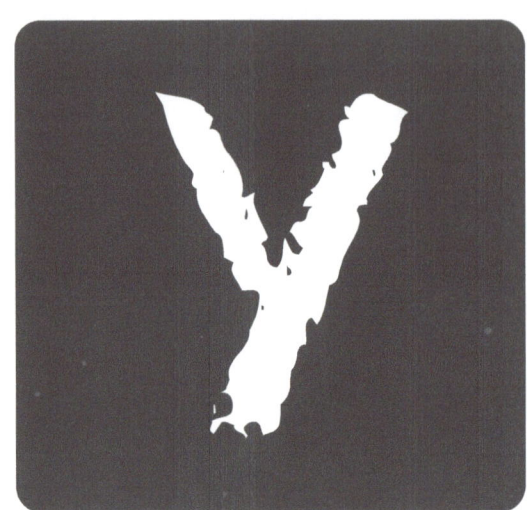

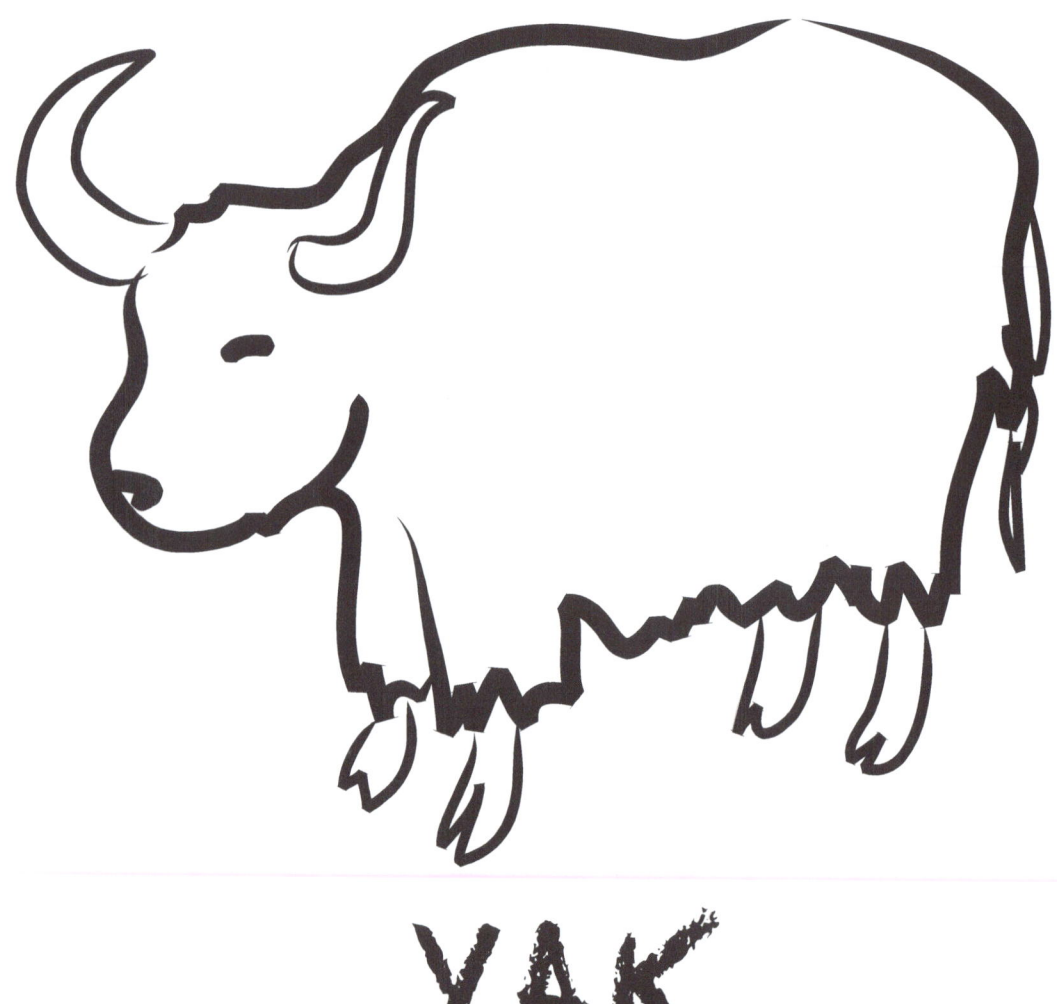

YAK

Get down on your hands and knees and lower your belly down to the floor.

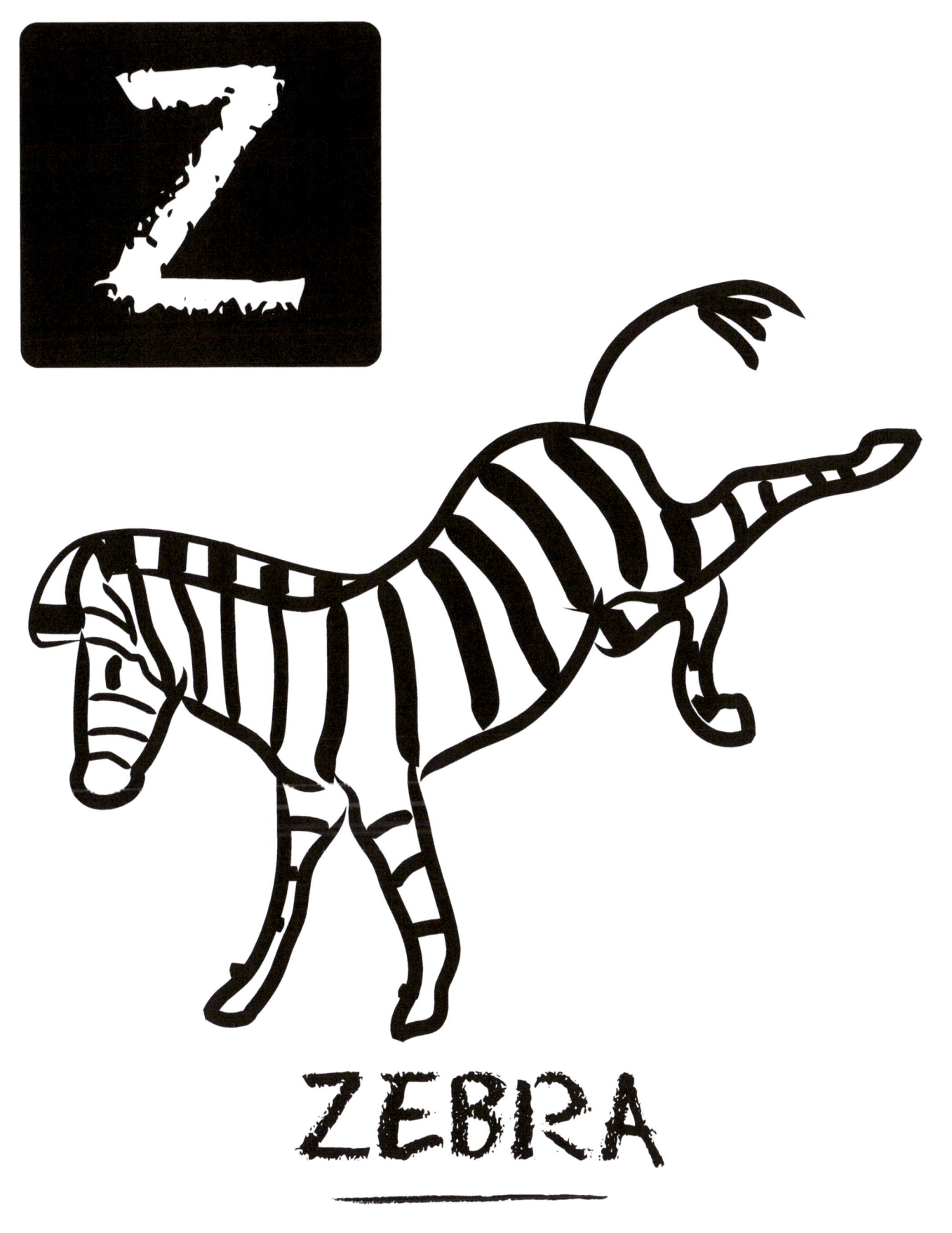

ZEBRA

Get down on your hands and knees and kick your legs up in the air behind you!

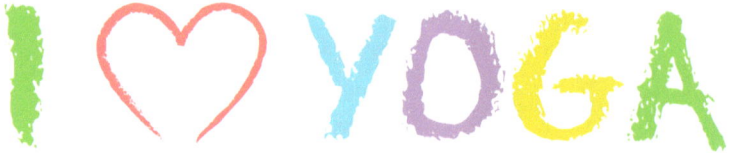

I ♥ YOGA

List 5 reasons you like yoga
and share one with your class!

I Like yoga because...

1. _____
_____

2. _____
_____

3. _____
_____

4. _____
_____

5. _____
_____

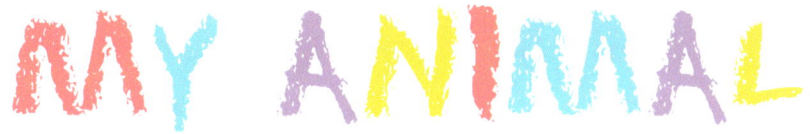

MY ANIMAL

Create your own animal! Use your imagination and draw a picture of an animal made up by you! Write down a description of your animal and give it a name. Then share it with your class and have your classmates figure out what kind of yoga pose your animal would have!

BALLOON BREATH

Imagine your belly is a balloon! Take long breaths in and out very slowly.
Let your belly balloon inflate and deflate as you breathe.
In which direction of breath did your balloon inflate?
In which direction did it deflate?

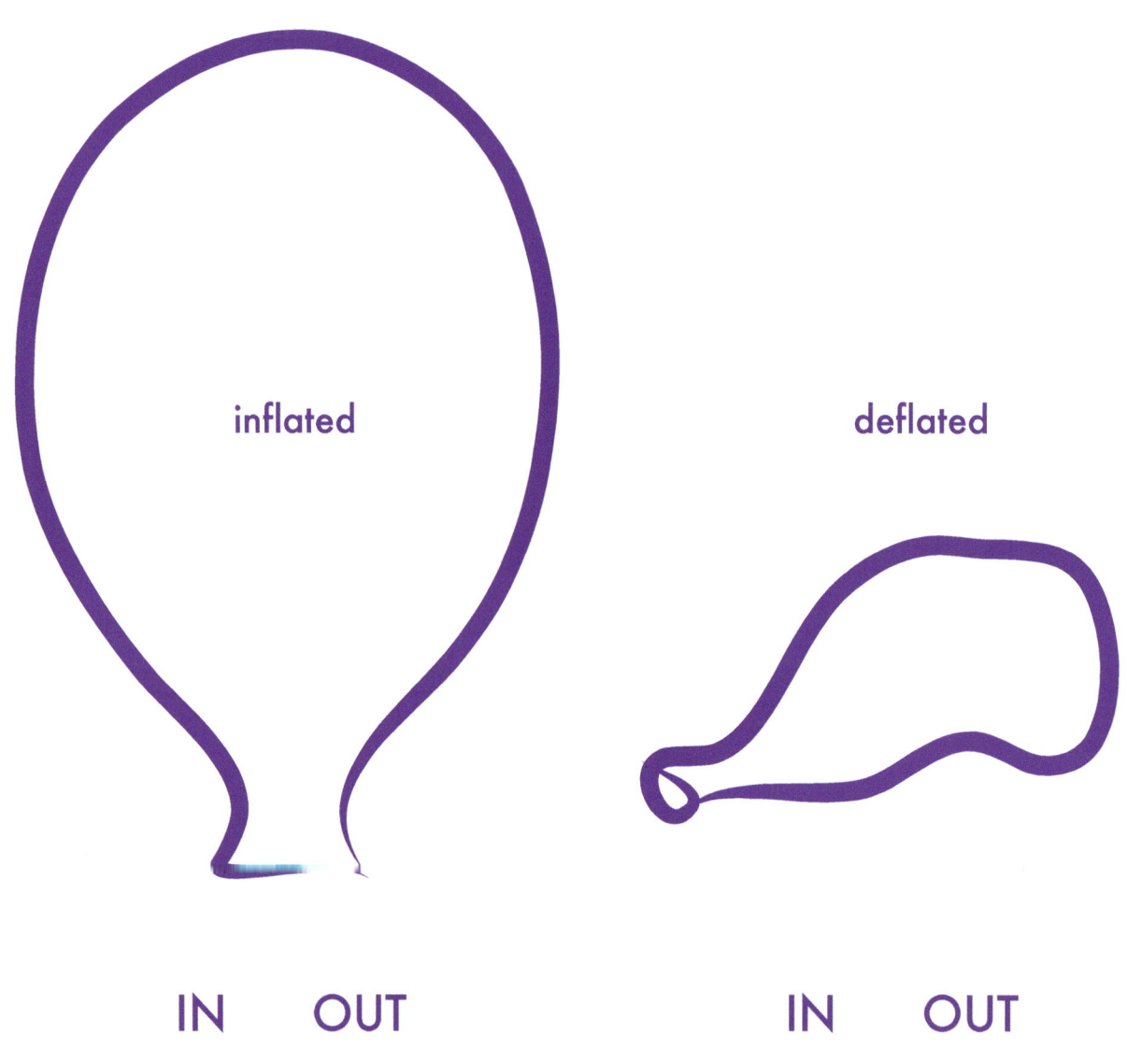

inflated

deflated

IN   OUT   IN   OUT

Circle the direction of breath that fits for each balloon.

STORYTIME YOGA

Draw a picture and write a story about your favorite animals!
Share the story with your class and use yoga poses to tell it!

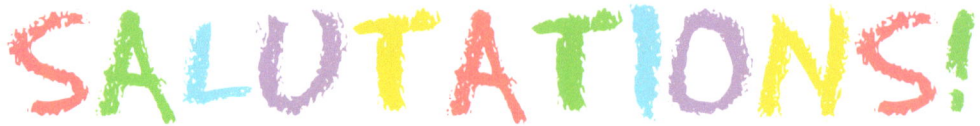

SALUTATIONS!

What is a Sun Salutation?

A Sun Salutation is a series of 12 poses performed in a single, graceful flow, like a dance. It is a way of saying hello to the sun. Work with your instructor on making a Sun Salutation and write down the sequence as you learn the poses!

1 _____

2 _____

3 _____

4 _____

5 _____

6 _____

7 _____

8 _____

9 _____

10 _____

11 _____

12 _____

Can you do the Sun Salutation without looking at the workbook? Give it a try!

YOU DID IT!

You did it! Congratulations on being an official Elahi Yoga student yogi or yogini! Write down the type of Elahi Yoga classmate you are and then write 5 reasonswhy you are proud of yourself!

I am a _____

I am proud of myself because...

1. _____
   _____

2. _____
   _____

3. _____
   _____

4. _____
   _____

5. _____
   _____

YOGA DICTIONARY

Asana - gentle stretching movements that help balance the mind and body.

Ashram - a secluded place where yoga and meditation are practiced.

Chakra - a center of radiating life force or energy.

Dhyana - meditation.

Drishti - the focus of the eyes in meditation.

Karma Yoga - yoga in which action is done as a duty, without any concern for success or failure.

Krlya - a traditional yoga purification movement that provides a cleansing process of one's inner body.

Mantra - a sacred mystic syllable, word or verse used in meditation to quiet the mind, and balance the inner body.

MedItatIon - the practice by which there is constant observation of the mind.

Mudra - a symbolic gesture transmitting or redirecting energy in yoga or meditation.

Namaste - a traditional Indian greeting of respect and thank you, with spiritual and symbol meaning.

Neti Neti - "Not this. Not this." Words you say when dismissing thoughts and sounds while meditating.

Om - a single-sound mantra that signifies the unification of the body, mind and spirit.

Padma - the sanskrit word for flower.

Prana - life energy, life force, or life current.

Sudhaka - a student who strives for a goal.

Shanti - is peace or tranquility in Sanskrit.

Sun Salutation - exercise that limbers up the whole body.

Ujjayi - loud breathing that involves drawing air in through both nostrils.

Vinyasa - yoga that means breathing and movement, is for internal cleansing.